POCKET GUIDE FOR STUDENTS

COMMUNITY PLACEMENTS

Pocket Guides for Student Nurses

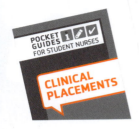

"A very useful, well-written and practical pocket book for any level of student nurse preparing for clinical placement. This book is also a great resource for lecturers and mentors to have, to help students get the most out of their placement time." ★★★★★

"This is such a useful guide that has just the right amount of need to know info for student nurses on clinical placement, as well as loads of little tips scattered throughout. A must-have for student nurses on placements!" ★★★★★

"Full of everything you need to know as a student nurse on placement. Written by students for students. Helpful little references to help with abbreviations and common medications. A must for any student about to head on placement." ★★★★★

Forthcoming titles in the series:

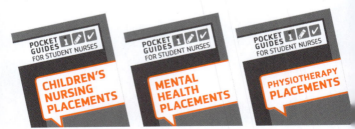

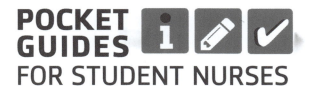

POCKET
GUIDES
FOR STUDENT NURSES

COMMUNITY
PLACEMENTS

**Lesley McKinlay, Georgios Tsigkas,
Caroline Dickson and Fiona Stuart**

*Queen Margaret University,
Edinburgh*

Lantern

ISBN: 9781908625557
First published in 2019 by Lantern Publishing Limited

Lantern Publishing Limited, The Old Hayloft, Vantage
Business Park, Bloxham Road, Banbury OX16 9UX, UK
www.lanternpublishing.com

British Library Cataloguing in Publication Data
A catalogue record for this book is available from the British Library

The authors and publisher have made every attempt to ensure
the content of this book is up to date and accurate. However,
healthcare knowledge and information is changing all the time
so the reader is advised to double-check any information in
this text on drug usage, treatment procedures, the use of
equipment, etc. to confirm that it complies with the latest safety
recommendations, standards of practice and legislation, as well as
local Trust policies and procedures. Students are advised to check
with their tutor and/or mentor before carrying out any of the
procedures in this textbook.

Typeset by Medlar Publishing Solutions Pvt Ltd, India
Printed and bound in the UK
Distributed by NBN International, 10 Thornbury Road,
Plymouth, PL6 7PP, UK

Last digit is the print number: 10 9 8 7 6 5 4 3 2 1

Personal information

Name: . . . .

Mobile: . . . .

Address during placement: . . . .

. . . .

. . . .

. . . .

PLACEMENT DETAILS

Practice location: . . . .

Practice address: . . . .

. . . .

. . . .

. . . .

CONTACT IN CASE OF EMERGENCY

Name: . . . .

Mobile: . . . .

Home/Work number: . . . .

Contents

Preface

We were invited to write this book to be part of the series of Pocket Guides for pre-registration student nurses across the UK. As with the *Clinical Placements* Pocket Guide, students were invited to participate. Two focus groups were held with pre-registration nursing students and students from the district nursing and health visiting programmes. Using the same format as the *Clinical Placements* Pocket Guide, we facilitated spaces where students were able to identify top tips relating to preparing for and being on community placement. Their energy and enthusiasm to engage with this was fantastic, despite the heavy workload generated by their studies. Students then formed small groups where pre- and post-registration students worked together to begin the writing process. As a group of lecturers, we have brought the students' contributions into the book format, building on the work they had begun. Finally, we sought feedback from the students to ensure the book reflected their intended outcomes. Critical readers with a community nursing background made comments on the final version.

We refer to 'mentors' as well as 'supervisors' throughout this book as the registered healthcare professionals who will be overseeing and assessing your community practice placement. When the new NMC standards framework for nursing and midwifery education (2018) are widely implemented, the mentoring system will change and we will update the advice in this Pocket Guide accordingly.

Lesley, Georgios, Caroline and Fiona

September 2018

Acknowledgements

We are grateful for contributions from students and hope that their experiences and advice are useful to other students. Special thanks go to Sara Moran-Winchester for her cartoon illustrations. Lastly, our thanks must go to Peter Oates from Lantern Publishing for his support during the writing process and his incredible patience.

Student contributors:

Tracy Maguire, Sara Moran-Winchester, Rebecca Paul, Anna Campbell, Emma Irvine, Aileen Cameron, Amanda Fairbairn, Marianne Ward.

The publishers would like to thank Kirstie Paterson and Jessica Wallar, authors of *Clinical Placements*, the first Pocket Guide in this series, and Kath MacDonald, their editor, for permission to use some of the content from their book as well as the overall framework.

Abbreviations

Recognised prescription abbreviations			
BD	twice daily	PR	per rectum
g	gram	PRN	when required
ID	intradermal	PV	per vagina
IM	intramuscular	QDS	four times daily
INH	inhaled	SC	subcutaneous
IV	intravenous	SL	sublingual
mg	milligram	stat	immediately
ml	millilitre	TDS	three times daily
OD	once a day	TOP	topical

Professionals	
CPN	Community Psychiatric Nurse
DN (SPDN)	District Nurse (Specialist Practitioner District Nurse)
GP	General Practitioner
HCA	Health Care Assistant
HCSW	Health Care Support Worker
OT	Occupational Therapist
PT/Physio	Physiotherapist
SCPHN	Specialist Community Public Health Nurse – School Nurse/Health Visitor/Occupational Health Nurse
SLT	Speech and Language Therapist
SW	Social Worker

Some commonly used abbreviations are listed below but the NMC Code (2015) recommends avoiding the use of unnecessary abbreviations.

Abbreviations can sometimes mean different things in different circumstances; e.g. OD in prescribing means 'once daily', whereas in other settings it can mean 'overdose'. It is for this reason that the NMC Code suggests avoiding the use of abbreviations.

BMI	body mass index
BP	blood pressure
CD	controlled drug
D&V	diarrhoea and vomiting
DNA	did not attend
DNACPR	do not attempt cardiopulmonary resuscitation
DOB	date of birth
HR	heart rate
MRSA	methicillin-resistant *Staphylococcus aureus*
MSSU	midstream specimen of urine
MUST	Malnutrition Universal Screening Tool
OD	overdose
OFC	occipitofrontal circumference
PMH	past medical history
PND	postnatal depression
RR	respiratory rate
SOB	shortness of breath
TPR	temperature, pulse, respiration
UTI	urinary tract infection

Getting there

1 Preparing for community placement

In the UK, health services are increasingly being delivered in primary care and community settings. A community setting will allow you to see health and social care across the lifespan. This means that you may have the opportunity to work with a variety of people, who offer various services based in the community area/primary care. Primary care is known as the 'front door' of healthcare and social services and it is often the first point of contact for patients. This may include care provision by GPs, community nurses, dentists and pharmacists.

Your placement area may be in a range of settings within primary care, for example:

- Health centres/medical practices (with District/Community Nurse, Health Visitor, School Nurse or Practice Nurse)
- Care or residential homes
- Community hospitals
- Charities (third sector organisations)
- Social work
- Education settings.

In preparation for your practice placement, you should contact a member of the community team to introduce yourself and make plans for commencing. Ideally, this should be arranged a week prior to your start date.

Use these questions to obtain the information you will need to prepare for your first visit to your placement area.

Preparation questions

- Who is my mentor?
- Should I wear my student nurse uniform?
- Where do I get changed?
- How do I get there?
- What is the best mode of transport / what is the parking situation?
- Where is the meeting point?
- What is the break schedule?
- How do I gain access to the community base area?
- What will be my working days / hours?
- Is there a staff canteen or can I get my lunch elsewhere?
- Is there a secure area where I can leave my personal belongings?

Notes

Do some research on the community in which your placement will take place. Find information about the area to make you aware of the community environment and population groups you may encounter. This is somewhere you will work for several weeks, so it is valuable to know what to expect.

✅ Checklist of things to bring with you on your first day

- ☐ *Student identification card*
- ☐ *Practice placement assessment documentation*
- ☐ *Spare uniform*
- ☐ *Water bottle*
- ☐ *Name badge (if you have one)*
- ☐ *Food and drink*
- ☐ *Notepad and pen*
- ☐ *Any questions you may have*

✏️ Notes

There will be a local uniform policy which you should familiarise yourself with. In the community you may not be required to wear uniform, but if that is the case, remember you are still representing the nursing profession and look smart.

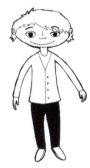

Smart student

Your responsibilities include:

- Hair should be tied back and off the collar (not necessary for health visiting).
- Nails should be short and clean with no nail varnish.
- No jewellery except wedding or other plain band.
- Wear name badge (see local policy).
- Wear a smart skirt or trousers.
- Footwear should be flat, clean, comfortable and closed toe.
- If providing direct clinical care, wear short-sleeved shirt/blouse/top (or sleeves rolled up so that arms are bare below the elbow) and avoid wearing neckties.

Your placement may have specific uniform requirements – note them here:

Absence policy

Ensure you are aware of the absence policies of the university and placement area. If you are absent, you must make sure both areas are informed prior to your start time. You may self-certify for seven days but if absent for longer than this, you will be required to submit a GP letter as evidence to your university contact. Prior to returning to practice, you should advise your mentor and university as per policy.

ℹ Top tip

Remember, messages left with receptionists may not reach your mentor in time for the start of your working day, so if possible, contact your mentor directly.

While you are on your community placement, you will be encouraged to shadow different health and social care professionals and visit a range of community-based services. You should always make your mentor aware of where you are. This is to ensure your safety.

ℹ Top tip

Share your mobile number with your mentor while you are on placement.

 Notes

_____

_____

_____

4.1 The NMC Code

All nurses, midwives and Health Visitors adhere to the Nursing and Midwifery Council (NMC) Code of Conduct. As a student, this also applies to you, so it is important you are familiar with its contents.

Read the Code at **bit.ly/NMC-Code**

To make it easy for you to access them, we have shortened web links to this format – simply type these into any web browser and you'll go to the right page!

The Code centres around four elements:

- Prioritising people
- Practising effectively
- Preserving safety
- Promoting professionalism and trust.

 Top tip

Discuss with your mentor how these elements are evidenced in a range of community settings, and write your thoughts here:

4.2 Raising concerns

If you witness any situation in your placement which you think puts a member of the public at risk, or if you have any concerns about the care or professionalism you see in practice, then you are responsible for reporting this to protect patient safety. You should abide by local policies, but first you need to talk to your mentor or university contact. You should find guidance in your practice assessment documentation, and the NMC also has guidance on raising concerns as a student at **bit.ly/NMC-RC1**, and as a nurse or midwife at **bit.ly/NMC-RC2**.

Top tip

Familiarise yourself with the local university and organisational policy around raising concerns and discuss this with your mentor.

Notes

4.3 Consent and confidentiality

Gaining consent and maintaining confidentiality within community settings are as important as in any setting. Ensuring verbal or written consent is gained, as appropriate, is an important aspect of the NMC Code. No procedures should be undertaken without the person's agreement. If a person is unable to give verbal or written consent, due to inability to make decisions for themselves or to communicate, then practitioners will refer to the appropriate Government Acts according to the country of practice.

- England and Wales: Mental Capacity Act: making decisions (2005)
- Scotland: Adults with Incapacity Act (2000)
- Northern Ireland: Mental Capacity Act (2016).

These Acts aim to protect people who cannot consent for themselves by allocating a welfare guardian to be part of the decision-making process and act in the person's best interest. Some examples where these may be useful are for a person with dementia, acquired brain injury or learning disabilities.

No procedure should ever be forced on a person, with or without them having capacity. If a person refuses care, then this should be documented and communicated to the necessary people. For a person without capacity who may not be able to make decisions or communicate them, the designated guardian has the legal right to make these decisions regarding consent. If this person is not available, then the visit and care procedure may have to be rescheduled.

Top tip

As a student nurse, always refer to your registered nurse mentor/supervisor for advice, and never give care that was not consented to. Consider ways to gain consent when caring for a baby or young child.

Normally, people over the age of 16 are entitled to consent to their own treatment. A person under the age of 16 may consent to their own treatment if they are believed to have capacity to understand and fully appreciate what is involved in their treatment. This means that they are competent to make their own decision. In England, this is called *Gillick competence* and there are variations of this in Scotland, Northern Ireland and Wales.

Maintaining confidentiality is an expectation of your professional behaviour. In your community placement, you will be in a variety of formal and informal settings. You may meet people in a professional context whom you know socially. Speak with your mentor, as it may be inappropriate for you to be involved in their care. You may also meet people socially whom you have met in a professional context. It is vital that you maintain confidentiality and the highest standards of professionalism; refer to the Code at **bit.ly/NMC-Code**.

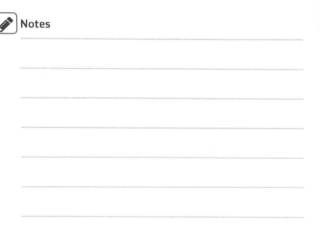 Notes

4.4 Social media

Healthcare professionals, nursing students and carers should use social media responsibly, respecting the privacy and confidentiality of patients at all times. Social media platforms can be used with care by healthcare professionals to share professional knowledge and network with colleagues. Community teams can find these particularly useful as they can be working remotely.

ℹ️ Tips for maintaining professionalism

- Do not write any posts about anyone in the professional context on an open Facebook platform.
- No aspect of a patient's care, including identification or setting, should be posted.
- Remember, even anonymised situations may be identifiable.
- In your professional capacity, do not interact with patients, relatives and carers on social media sites.
- Do not use discriminatory language.
- Do not bully, intimidate or exploit people online.
- Do not post pictures of patients or the practice placement area.

The NMC has published guidelines for using social media responsibly, which you can find here: **bit.ly/NMC-SM**

 Notes

Person-centred practice

As healthcare professionals, we should be person-centred in the way we interact with patients, families and each other. You will hear the terms *person-centred care* and *person-centred practice* (PCP). McCormack and McCance (2017) have produced a framework that identifies outcomes of PCP, the ways of achieving this and environments that encourage this way of being.

The home environment lends itself well to PCP and you should observe how your mentor and other practitioners form relationships with their patients or people in their care and how they reach shared decisions. You can begin to be person-centred by talking to patients and families about what it is like to be supported and cared for in your practice area. Try to find out what is important to them and discuss with your mentor how you can develop McCormack and McCance's care processes.

Top tip

A reflective diary is a useful tool to help you make sense of your learning experiences. You will have discussed reflective models in university and you will find them useful to help you learn from your practice for future use. When reflecting, consider how your or others' practice reflects the Person-centred Practice Framework. This may be useful for future academic assignments and completion of your personal portfolio.

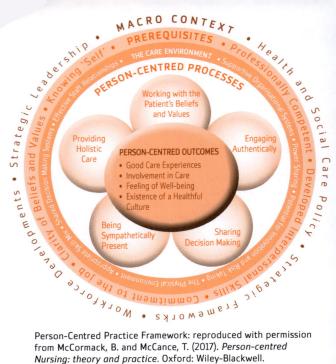

Person-Centred Practice Framework: reproduced with permission from McCormack, B. and McCance, T. (2017). *Person-centred Nursing: theory and practice*. Oxford: Wiley-Blackwell.

✏️ **Notes**

_____

_____

_____

Settling there

Tips for your first day

- Make sure you arrive on time and go to the agreed place to meet your mentor.
- Introduce yourself and wear your badge/ID.
- You should be introduced to relevant members of the team and be shown around your placement area.
- Familiarise yourself with the community base.
- Discuss with your mentor the health and safety requirements (e.g. in event of a fire).
- Clarify the working shift pattern (if appropriate), as these can be different depending on which locality you are working in.
- Use your mobile phone for professional reasons only.
- Keep a diary of your activities, thoughts and feelings. This can help ensure that you are achieving your learning outcomes and may inform discussions with your mentor or clinical supervisor.

Note here important names and contact details of your colleagues. Consider their roles and responsibilities.

Key colleagues you will be working with

Nursing in the community focuses on health and the causes of ill health in the broadest sense. These are known as the determinants of health. Nurses and other members of the multidisciplinary team consider the impact of the physical, emotional and social setting on individuals and their families in their assessments.

Rather than being illness- or problem-focused, community nurses take a strengths-based approach to health and wellbeing. This means they help service users identify and focus on things they *can* do, rather than things they can't. As part of this approach, community nurses support individuals, families and groups to access resources within their community. It is important the community nurse has access to a community profile (see *Section 8* on getting to know your community). Terminology such as health education and promotion, self-care and self-management are used by all health and social care professionals.

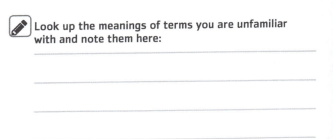 **Look up the meanings of terms you are unfamiliar with and note them here:**

✏️ **Notes**

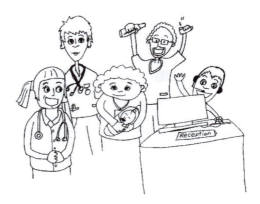

The multidisciplinary team.

Your mentor / supervisor is likely to be a SCPHN, SPDN or General Practice Nurse.

7.1 Health Visitors

All Health Visitors (HV) are registered nurses or midwives with an additional registration in Specialist Community Public Health Nursing (SCPHN). The role of the Health Visitor is to promote positive health and wellbeing outcomes for children (usually between birth and 5 years old), their families and the community. You may observe clinics, where children have developmental checks or immunisations. You will also accompany the Health Visitor on home visits.

A particular focus of a Health Visitor is working with vulnerable families. The majority of families receive a universal service via home visits and can access child drop-in clinics for information, support and developmental reviews. However, some families require further interventions and support with aspects such as mental health, developmental needs and children with long-term health issues.

An important aspect of the HV role involves working with other organisations to safeguard and protect children. Assessing and recognising risk and signs of abuse or neglect are essential skills. You may observe some of the work related to this if it is appropriate for you to be involved.

Health Visitors may also work with at-risk or deprived groups which may include travellers, people with addiction issues and the homeless.

Other roles may include:
- Providing antenatal and postnatal support
- Supporting children with special needs
- Giving advice on feeding babies and children
- Monitoring child development and addressing any needs of the child
- Advising on behavioural management techniques
- Risk assessing and aiming to reduce accidents and injuries to children.

7.2 District Nurses

District Nurses lead teams of nurses and healthcare support workers to deliver care to patients, normally in a patient's own home. Normally, they have an additional professional qualification that is recorded on the NMC register. This is a Specialist Practitioner Qualification. They manage a caseload of patients and lead a team. Patients on the caseload often have one or more long-term conditions, may be frail, older people and/or at the end of their life.

The aim of care provided is to avoid patients having to go into hospital unnecessarily, and DNs do this by coordinating care delivered by a range of health and social care professionals. They are also skilled in anticipating patients' care needs, which means they can put things in place to help patients and families participate in decisions about, and manage, their own care. DNs also manage budgets and other resources, and develop their team, ensuring everyone is competent, continually developing and feels supported. Some DNs are advanced practitioners who can prescribe medicines for patients on their caseload.

7.3 General Practice Nurses

General Practice Nurses normally work in the GP practice, promoting health and wellbeing to people across the lifespan. The focus of their role is in the main preventative, and includes supporting people to manage their long-term conditions, travel health, women's health and sometimes treatment room activities. People would come to the treatment room if they required medication they were unable to administer themselves, had a wound they needed dressed or for treatment of minor injuries and illness. Some people attend the treatment room in an emergency situation, e.g. deterioration of their asthma or other respiratory conditions, anaphylaxis or trauma.

7.4 School Nurses

You may have a placement or part-placement with a school nurse. They are qualified and registered practitioners (nurses or midwives), many of whom have chosen to gain an additional qualification to become a Specialist Community Public Health Nurse (SCPHN). They support children and young people to make healthy life choices, enabling them to enjoy a healthy and fulfilling life. School nurses work across the education and healthcare sectors, providing a link between school, home and the community.

Tips on observing practice

Notice strengths-based approaches used by different professionals to help individuals, families and groups maximise their own health, and discuss these with your mentor.

There will be a number of different agencies involved in community health and social care within your placement area. In discussion with your mentor, you may wish to explore these services and arrange visits as appropriate.

Top tip

Take the opportunity to shadow as many members of the multidisciplinary team as you can and record their roles and responsibilities below.

Useful resources

For information on exploring and transitioning to different nursing roles: bit.ly/QNI-info and bit.ly/NHS-roles

Notes

8

Getting to know your community

Community profiling helps you gain an understanding of the area you are working in. This will include health needs and services available. Voluntary services are an excellent way of getting to know the area you are visiting on placement. You may wish to get in touch with them to arrange to spend some time with such organisations, and see how they are relevant to your assigned area.

For example:

- Breastfeeding support groups, new father groups and young parent support groups link closely with the Health Visiting team to support new families.
- Day centres, support groups and befriending services may be in place to combat social isolation; this is an important part of providing holistic care.
- Additionally, District Nursing palliative care support is often assisted by third sector organisations, such as Macmillan, Marie Curie or a local hospice.

Spending time working with staff from these organisations may help you achieve some of the learning outcomes for your practice placement.

Notes

_____

_____

_____

_____

i **Tips on getting to know your community**

Get to know your community by walking, cycling or driving around and use your senses to notice what it is like to live here.

- What types of housing do you see? Are there any green spaces or areas of disrepair?
- What facilities are there in terms of shops, banks, schools, social/leisure opportunities and public transport?
- What noises do you hear? Think about industries, traffic and noises of nature.
- What can you smell? Are there pleasant smells, or those that are present as a by-product of industry?
- Compare what you notice with the community profile available in your placement area.

🖊 **Notes**

_____

_____

_____

_____

_____

_____

_____

Your mentor/supervisor will work with you to plan your learning activities that will enable you to meet the learning outcomes for your practice placement. Take time to discuss with them the potential learning opportunities, and make a plan together.

Points to consider:

- Agree ways of working with your mentor.
- Identify how your mentor will support you in achieving these objectives.
- Find out how and when your ongoing achievement records will be signed off.
- Identify a way that you can alert your mentor to a situation that you feel unsafe or unhappy with.
- There may be some visits that you are unable to attend or times when there is less for you to be involved with. Check with your mentor how this will be decided and communicated to you so that you can organise an alternative activity.
- You may wish to share with your mentor any specific health issue or learning need.

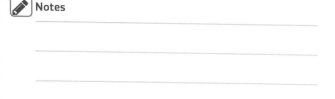 **Notes**

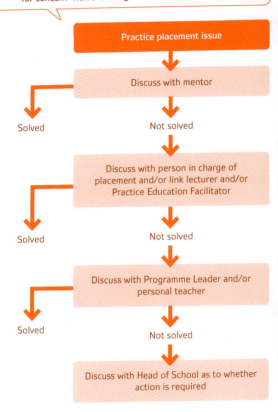

If you are concerned about your supervision or any other aspect of your experience, discuss this with your academic link. The university will have a process for addressing this – a simple "cause for concern" flowchart might look something like this:

Practice placement issue

Discuss with mentor

Solved

Not solved

Discuss with person in charge of placement and/or link lecturer and/or Practice Education Facilitator

Solved

Not solved

Discuss with Programme Leader and/or personal teacher

Solved

Not solved

Discuss with Head of School as to whether action is required

Being there

You should prepare yourself for a home visit by finding out as much as you can about the patient or family. It is good to be proactive but you should always be guided by your mentor or the practitioner you are working with.

Tips for preparing for a visit

- Access paper or electronic records, as appropriate.
- Determine your role during the visit (are you observing or will you be expected to participate actively?).
- Consider how you will overcome any communication barriers, e.g. if the person is deaf, blind or if English is not their first language.
- Consider what equipment you may need, e.g. weighing scales, charts, dressing packs, syringes, needles, gloves, aprons, alcohol gel. This will vary depending on the type of visit.
- Find out from your mentor/supervisor the appropriate mode of accessing the home.
- Gain permission to access a key safe, if applicable. Your mentor/supervisor may familiarise you with the keypad system.

Entering someone's home

Remember you are a guest in a person's home so you need to ask permission to enter and to carry out procedures. You must respect the person's home environment.

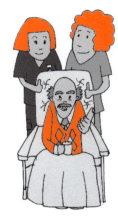

Tips during a home visit

- Remember to introduce yourself to the person.
- Make conversation – it is important to establish a relationship with the person so that they feel comfortable with you.
- Request pets to be moved to another room if appropriate.
- Look about you at the person's surroundings and think about the environment. This may include heating and any potential hazards.
- Observe interactions between the person and their families/carers or parents and babies/young children.
- Respect the person's way of living; however, if you identify any particular risk you should discuss this with your mentor/supervisor.

- Listen actively – focus on the person and acknowledge that you have heard them and they have understood the discussion.
- Provide the person with an opportunity to ask questions.
- Ensure a suitable arrangement is made for any necessary future visit.
- Ensure you leave the house as the person wishes and if appropriate, return the key to the key safe.

Notes

Interpersonal skills are central to everything that nurses do. Effective communication can make a positive difference to a person or their relatives. Remember you may be the only person that has visited that day.

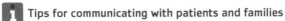 **Tips for communicating with patients and families**

- Introduce yourself with your name and title.
- Ask the person how they would like to be addressed.
- Always explain the purpose of your visit and give relevant information about the situation.
- Take into consideration if the person has communication problems, such as poor eyesight or hearing difficulties. Consider ways which will make communication easier (e.g. ensure glasses / hearing aids are in place, as appropriate).
- Ensure you show interest with good eye contact.
- Be clear and ensure the person can understand you; do not use jargon.
- You may see, hear or smell things which may make you feel uncomfortable. Think about how you react and be aware of your own body language.
- Observe the person's non-verbal communication and what this might mean.
- Offer the person an opportunity to ask questions and voice any concerns.
- Actively listen to the person and clarify understanding by summarising or paraphrasing key points.
- Consider an appropriate place within the home which may be free from distraction.
- Always be honest and remember to say "I don't know but I will find out" if required.

Notes

Working closely with the wider multidisciplinary and multi-agency teams is part of community working. Shared care or joint visits are common in the community so that holistic care can be provided to the person and a good care experience can be achieved.

During your placement, you will be communicating with a range of different professionals and support staff. Effective communication is essential to ensure high quality and efficient services. As a student nurse, you may not be confident with this aspect of the role and may not have previous experience of these situations. However, you should use your practice placement experience to observe, listen, interact and learn with your mentor/supervisor and identify ways of being involved to develop your communication skills.

12.1 Nursing handover

Most nursing teams have a 'handover' to discuss patients they have visited. This normally occurs in the health centre/clinic. Many teams use a framework such as SBAR

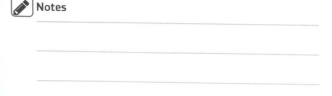

Notes

to hand over and this is a good opportunity to practise, to build up confidence when presenting patients. When you feel confident, ask to present one or two patients that you and your mentor / supervisor may have visited during the day. Communication is a skill which improves the more you do it. Do not be afraid to ask for help and advice. A good way to learn is to listen to how others do it. If you are not sure of something, take the time to stop and ask.

Top tip

It is worth making a few notes identifying what you think the team needs to know in a handover. Presenting patients will get easier once you have done it a few times.

The SBAR framework is often used in practice. It can be used effectively to escalate a clinical problem that requires immediate attention, or to facilitate efficient handover. This is more commonly used in hospital settings but is becoming increasingly utilised in community settings.

Situation	Identify yourself and the area you are calling from
	Identify the patient by name and the reason for calling
	Describe your concern
Background	Give a short patient history, including diagnosis and relevant medication
	Explain what happened
Assessment	Vital signs
	Concerns, e.g. description of a wound
Recommendation	Explain what you need – be specific
	Make suggestions
	Clarify your and the patient's expectations

Example of an SBAR handover:

Situation	Hello, my name is Lucy, a student nurse working with an SPDN. We visited Mrs Smith today who lives in Cairney Lane; her date of birth is 12.03.32. We are concerned she has a wound infection.
Background	Mrs Smith has a leg ulcer on the anterior aspect of her left leg. She has had this for a few weeks, after knocking it on her table, and it has been healing well until now. She is housebound due to mobility problems, she has type 2 diabetes which is well controlled, she has no known allergies.
Assessment	On assessment it was noticed that the exudate from her wound has increased and is now green in colour, there is a malodour and she is experiencing more pain around the area. The tissue around the wound is inflamed and red and her observations are all within normal parameters with the exception of a temperature of 38°C. We have taken a wound swab and applied an antibacterial dressing.
Recommendation	A wound swab has been sent to the microbiology laboratory. The results will determine if infection is present and an appropriate antibiotic can be prescribed if necessary. Wound assessment and dressing changes will be documented in a wound chart.

12.2 Answering the telephone

This may be an anxiety-provoking task but the more you do it, the easier it will become. It may be an excellent way to support and help the nursing team, especially during busy times.

ℹ️ Tips on answering the phone

- Check with the team as to when the phone should be answered (some teams prefer it not to be answered during handover).
- Check if the messages are written down in a particular place, e.g. a diary.
- State your name, title and location.
- Ask "What can I help you with?"
- Write down the particulars, e.g. the caller's name, address and telephone number and what the concern / question is.
- Do not disclose any information regarding patients.
- If you need to ask a colleague's advice, tell the person you will be putting them on hold, and mute the call before discussing the situation.
- Ensure you hand the information over to a member of the nursing team if it cannot be dealt with there and then.
- If you are not in a position to answer questions, state that you are a student nurse and pass the phone to an available member of the team. If this is not possible, make sure you take details of the caller with a contact number and ensure follow-up at a later time.

Example of a phone call:

- "Good morning, community nurses' phone, Lucy the student nurse speaking."
- "How can I help you?"
- "Can you please confirm your name, address and date of birth?"

- "Mrs Smith, how can I help you today?"
- "The community nurse is unable to speak to you at present. Can I take a message and they will get back to you this afternoon/tomorrow/this week?"
- "Please can you give me a telephone number where we can contact you? Let me repeat that back to make sure I have heard you correctly."
- "Is there anything else I can help you with?"
- "Thank you and goodbye."

✎ **Notes**

_____

_____

_____

_____

_____

_____

_____

_____

_____

_____

Health and safety is just as important in the community/home setting as it is in a hospital environment. Procedures may differ depending on the role of the healthcare professional and local policy.

Some aspects of health and safety to think about include:

- Infection control
- Manual handling/moving and handling
- Lone working policy
- Violence and aggression.

13.1 Infection control

Effective hand hygiene is the key intervention which will prevent the spread of infection. The diagram below shows the recommended hand hygiene procedure.

You may be issued with pocket hand gel to be used during clinical procedures as per local policy. Certain interventions such as wound dressings and catheterisations will require a sterile procedure. Disposable equipment can be taken to

Notes

_____

_____

_____

_____

_____

the home and the cleanest available surface should be used to open any sterile packs. You may need to request space to be made. It is not advisable to use the floor, if this can be avoided. If there are pets which may contaminate sterile equipment, then it should be requested that the animal(s) be moved to another room or area if possible.

RUB HANDS FOR HAND HYGIENE! WASH HANDS WHEN VISIBLY SOILED

Duration of the entire procedure: 20-30 seconds

Apply a palmful of the product in a cupped hand, covering all surfaces;

Rub hands palm to palm;

Right palm over left dorsum with interlaced fingers and vice versa;

Palm to palm with fingers interlaced;

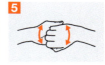

Backs of fingers to opposing palms with fingers interlocked;

Rotational rubbing of left thumb clasped in right palm and vice versa;

Rotational rubbing, backwards and forwards with clasped fingers of right hand in left palm and vice versa;

Once dry, your hands are safe.

Proper hand rub technique (World Health Organization, 2009). Reproduced with permission of the World Health Organization, www.who.int.

There will be local policies for clinical waste, with which you should familiarise yourself. If sharps are to be used within a home environment, appropriate arrangements should be made for the provision of a sharps bin and suitable plans made for the disposal of this when necessary.

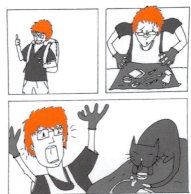

Keep pets and patients apart during your visit!

13.2 Manual handling

All healthcare professionals, including students, should have appropriate manual handling training (you might also come across the term 'moving and handling'). It is important to adopt safe manual handling practices in the community area to reduce any risk of injury to the healthcare professional or to the person.

Not all houses are adapted for disabled access and this can present challenges to safe manual handling in the community setting. When there are circumstances to overcome, in order to keep a person in their own home, there will often be a multidisciplinary approach and shared decision-making with the person and their family/carers.

Community nurses may have to be involved with the organisation of getting hospital beds/special mattresses into people's homes, electronic hoists for ease of moving patients, commode chairs for toileting access if a bathroom cannot be reached, and other specialised equipment such as glide sheets and pillow elevators to aid the moving of a person within the home.

Notes

13.3 Lone working

Many community nurses are often required to work alone and this can potentially pose a risk to their safety. As a student nurse, you will usually be working with your supervisor / mentor or another experienced care professional. It is unlikely that you will be asked to work independently.

Each member of the team should share their planned visits and locations with colleagues, to assure personal safety. Lone working policies exist within local areas and should be followed in any aspect of care. You should also check university policies in relation to lone working in your community placement. It is a safe practice to have a mobile phone available, which may be supplied to you in certain areas. You should ensure that you have shared relevant numbers with your supervisor / mentor.

Key points to consider in the unlikely event of you visiting alone:

- What is my risk assessment? Risk assessments should be carried out before any care interventions.
- Do I need any further assessment from a member of the multidisciplinary team (e.g. physiotherapist)?
- Is the environment safe?
- Do I need to move any furniture / equipment to make the environment safe? (consent is required)
- How can I ensure dignity is maintained?
- Have I communicated appropriately with the person / family?
- Is all the necessary equipment available?
- Can I carry out this task alone?
- Am I confident with what I am doing? Do I need advice from my supervisor / mentor?
- Do I know who to contact, should there be an adverse event?

Top tip

If ever you feel uncomfortable about carrying out a home visit, you should discuss this with your supervisor/mentor.

Notes

_____

_____

_____

_____

_____

_____

_____

_____

_____

_____

_____

_____

_____

_____

_____

There are many potential emergency situations which may occur in any community setting and some common examples are given below. Safety should be a priority for yourself firstly, and then for others.

ℹ Top tip

> As you are unlikely to have a team of healthcare professionals immediately available as you might have in hospital, you must be aware of the local procedures to follow in the event of an emergency or crisis situation.

14.1 Falls in the community

Frail older people are more likely to experience falls. This can result in serious injury and loss of confidence. There are teams in the community who respond quickly to help someone when they fall, rather than involving emergency services. Many people wear an alarm so they can call for help if they are unable to get up or are hurt. If you encounter someone who has fallen and you are not with an experienced practitioner, you should call for help and administer first aid. Discuss with your mentor when you would contact them, the GP, social services or dial 999.

There are also falls prevention teams, but every nurse should be assessing falls risk as part of their routine care and be aware of referral pathways. You can find out more by accessing the NICE falls pathway at **bit.ly/NICE-Falls**.

14.2 Infections and the risk of sepsis

Sepsis is a serious complication of an infection which can lead to multiple organ failure and death. Some common infections can cause sepsis, therefore it is important to recognise signs of infection and treat as necessary. Urinary tract infection, chest infection and wound infection are amongst the most prevalent causes of sepsis.

Sepsis can affect anyone, but children and older people may be particularly susceptible. You should be aware of the signs and symptoms, as sepsis must be diagnosed and treated as soon as possible. For more information visit **bit.ly/NHS-Sepsis**.

Other emergencies which could occur in the community include:

- Hypoglycaemia
- Myocardial infarction
- Anaphylaxis
- Stroke.

Your mentor/supervisor will assess the person and if there is concern for the person's safety, emergency services should be called and hospital transfer arranged if necessary. If you cannot gain access to someone's home and you can see that the person has collapsed or is injured, call the emergency services immediately.

Sometimes, there can be urgent or emergency situations relating to child protection and safeguarding, or a crisis at home situation which requires immediate attention. You will be guided by your mentor/supervisor and they will explain the processes and referrals required in individual cases.

ℹ️ Top tip

Remember you are not working alone; if you are faced with anything you are unsure about, discuss this with your mentor or another registered professional.

14.3 Basic Life Support (BLS)

If you come across an unresponsive person in your community placement, you should assess the situation for your own safety first and then intervene. Never do anything that you are not confident of or that puts your own safety at risk.

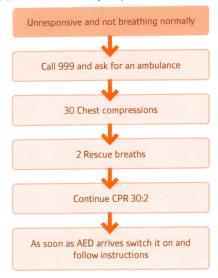

Adult Basic Life Support (Resuscitation Council, 2015).
CPR 30:2 – an emergency cardiopulmonary resuscitation procedure that alternates 30 chest compressions with two rescue breaths; AED – automated external defibrillator (a portable device that checks the heart rhythm and can send an electric shock to the heart to try to restore a normal rhythm). Reproduced with the kind permission of the Resuscitation Council (UK).

For infants and children, there are paediatric basic life support guidelines at **bit.ly/Resus-1**.

14.4 Violence and aggression

It is important to keep yourself safe and, where possible, not enter situations which are potentially dangerous. The community team will have carried out a risk assessment and if there is a known danger, then your mentor/supervisor should alert you. However, situations can be unpredictable. Remember to follow local policies and guidelines regarding lone working. You may have received training on dealing with violence and aggression/de-escalation techniques, and it may be useful in certain circumstances to use some of these to minimise risk within community areas.

Notes

It is essential that all care in any aspect of community nursing is documented accurately, in line with the NMC Code. Documentation will vary and care plans may have different formats. In the community, most documentation is multidisciplinary and available in paper and electronic formats. This may be linked to the GP records system, or professionals may have to record in both systems.

The documentation often used by Health Visitors includes:

- Child health records that include height and weight and growth charts – these are normally held by parents and recorded electronically
- Progress notes
- Child health surveillance programme – for developmental assessments
- Cause for concern records
- Immunisation records.

District nursing teams also use paper and electronic documentation systems which may be linked to social care. These are all tools that support District Nurses' assessment and care planning. Examples include:

- Single shared assessment
- Prescription sheet – states the prescribed drug, including dose, route and time, and is individual to each patient
- Waterlow Scale for identification of pressure sore risk (see inside back cover)
- Wound chart – identifies the initial wound assessment, wound measurements, management plan with dressing of choice, rationale and progress

- Malnutrition Universal Screening Tool (MUST) – assesses patients at risk of malnutrition or obesity (available at **bit.ly/MUST-BAPEN**)
- National Early Warning Score (NEWS) – a recognised standardised method for documenting patients' vital signs and advised action, which would be used if appropriate (see inside front cover, where it is reproduced from: Royal College of Physicians. *National Early Warning Score (NEWS) 2: Standardising the assessment of acute-illness severity in the NHS*. Updated report of a working party. London: RCP, 2017.)
- Care plan documenting the plan, progress and evaluation of care.

General Practice Nurses tend to document their care in the GP records. They may use some of the documentation outlined above.

Top tip

Familiarise yourself with the common documentation on placement; this may be available online.

Notes

_____

_____

_____

_____

_____

15.1 Incident reporting

If you are involved in an incident or near miss then it is important that appropriate documentation is completed for reporting this. Local policies for incident reporting must be followed. Datix is the software commonly used within the NHS. By reporting incidents and near misses, trends can be noted and action plans put in place to address any issues. The aim of incident reporting is to improve quality of care and reduce risk to patients. Typical incidents include:

- Drug administration error or near miss
- Equipment malfunction (medication pump or hoist)
- Witnessing an aggressive situation – person displaying aggressive behaviour towards a healthcare professional
- Person falling in the house during your visit
- An accident involving a young child or baby.

It is also important to be open and honest with patients/families, which is called duty of candour. More information around this can be found at **bit.ly/NMC-GMC**.

 Top tip

> Speak with your mentor/supervisor about how to complete local paperwork.

15.2 Yellow Card Scheme

The Yellow Card Scheme is vital in helping to monitor the safety of medicines and medical devices. If a patient experiences unanticipated side-effects of a medicine, or if there is a defect in a medical device, these should be reported to the Medicines and Healthcare products Regulatory Agency (MHRA) in the UK. The aim of this scheme is to ensure patient safety. Members of the public or healthcare professionals can alert the MHRA by completing the yellow form at the back of the British National Formulary (BNF) or online at yellowcard.mhra.gov.uk/. Reports can be made for all medicines including vaccines.

✎ Notes

Caring and supporting people across the lifespan

All professionals working in the community have a role in assessing a variety of health needs of individuals, families and the wider community across the lifespan. Their aim is promoting good health and preventing illness. You will be involved in childhood development, supporting people with long-term conditions and people with palliative and end of life care needs.

16.1 Childhood development

Child development begins prenatally and you will be able to observe antenatal and postnatal support with midwives, Health Visitors and nursery nurses. Health Visitors also have a role in providing advice on feeding babies and children and helping parents of young children develop parenting skills to give children the best start in life. They assess the growth and development of young children, with a particular focus on those with special needs. Your mentor / supervisor will support you with understanding the expected growth and development of children at various stages and how progress is monitored and documented.

16.2 Long-term conditions

Common long-term conditions include, but are not limited to, chronic obstructive pulmonary disease (COPD), heart failure, diabetes, multiple sclerosis (MS) and cancer. Healthcare professionals provide supportive family care as part of person-centred practice, as often family are the main carers for patients and look after them most of the time.

Many people are now living with long-term conditions in the community. Often they have two or three conditions, known as multimorbidities. The role of the health professional is to help people manage their condition themselves as much as possible and help keep them out of hospital. They do this by helping people to set goals that are important to them, through health promotion and anticipatory care. They also liaise with specialist services and colleagues from social services – this is called integrated working.

Promoting independence and helping people with long-term conditions to live at home involves arranging care, support and equipment to allow the person maximum ability to mobilise and carry out activities of their daily life as appropriate.

16.3 Palliative and end of life care

Being a part of the care team for a person who wishes to die at home is a privilege but you may find this a bit daunting, especially if you have no previous experience of death or looking after a dying person. It is natural to feel anxious about this aspect of care but you should always be well supported to learn and develop the necessary skills required in relation to palliative and end of life care.

District Nurses in particular are often involved with a person, their family and their extended network in the lead up to the end of someone's life. You may be involved in these support visits and will be able to observe how therapeutic relationships are developed.

As a person enters the final stages of life, the District Nurse has a role in keeping them as comfortable as possible. They will be involved in providing holistic care, including emotional care and support, personal care, and pain and symptom relief.

Palliative care relates to symptom control and promoting comfort for people with long-term conditions which will not be cured. Patients are often taking a variety of medicines to relieve their symptoms, which may include pain, sickness, agitation and difficulty breathing. Medication can be administered using a number of different routes, and you may witness administration of medicines via a syringe driver pump which gives medication subcutaneously continually over 24 hours.

The term 'end of life' is often used for the last year of someone's life. As a person reaches this stage, they may sleep much of the time and begin to lose consciousness, although this is not necessarily the case. The priority for caring for a dying person in the home is to keep them comfortable and as symptom-free as possible. It may also be important to them to have certain wishes granted, such as who is present with them. The healthcare professional can work with the family to try to fulfil these wishes.

16.4 Following a death in the community

When someone dies in the community, the death must be verified. This means carrying out certain checks to ensure the person has passed away and a form must be completed to state this. The healthcare professional who can verify a death must have had specific training and this is usually a doctor or registered nurse.

If the nurse is present then they will carry out last offices (final act of care) which means laying out the body if possible and ensuring the person is lying flat, is clean, has eyes and mouth closed and their dignity is maintained. Arrangements are then made to contact a funeral director who will arrange the removal of the person's body to a mortuary. During this process the nurse will be supporting the family and/or carers.

You may have personal experiences of death and dying and it is important to care for yourself. You may find it supportive to let your mentor know if you are struggling with any aspect of this. It will also be important for you to understand the aim, intended outcome and your role during the visit. You should also take time to reflect with your mentor/supervisor and it is natural and acceptable to feel upset.

Top tip

There are many healthcare strategies focusing on palliative and end of life care, so find out what is relevant to your area. There are also charities such as Marie Curie and local hospices who can offer practical advice and support, leaflets, sitting services and patient/carer support, so it is worth asking your mentor/supervisor for further information.

Notes

There are many healthcare professionals based within health centres, such as treatment room nurses, podiatrists, GPs, school nurses and midwives. You may find it useful and interesting to arrange to spend some time with other members of the multidisciplinary team. You may consider how the roles of the different healthcare professionals impact on care delivery within the community. Remember you will have to plan this in advance, so discuss suitable times and dates with your mentor and ask their advice about who to contact.

Top tip

Take your practice assessment documentation with you as it may be appropriate to update it during your visits. Set learning objectives and think about any questions you may have.

Notes

17.1 Practice assessment documentation

Throughout your practice placement, it is important to liaise with your mentor/supervisor and update your practice assessment documentation as you progress. Often there will be a midway assessment, which you should ensure is completed appropriately and on time.

Top tip

If you have any issues relating to your practice placement then make sure you discuss them with your mentor or academic link person as soon as possible.

Notes

_____

_____

_____

_____

_____

_____

_____

_____

_____

Moving on from there

Throughout your placement you will have been writing in your reflective diary or blog. This will enhance your learning and will include positive experiences and challenges you have faced. By critically reflecting, you will be able to consider how this may influence your future practice. The reflective process can be carried out in different ways and some examples are shown below.

Unstructured reflection methods

- Note taking
- Keeping a reflective diary/portfolio
- Informal dialogue with peers, colleagues, mentor.

Structured reflection methods

- Group supervision meetings led by a facilitator
- Reflective essay writing
- Using a reflective model to structure the process.

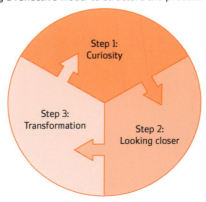

The 3-stage (CLT) model of reflection.

Reflection is essential for developing and being the best you can be:

- Reflect on what went well
- Reflect on what didn't go well
- Reflect on how you felt
- Make an action plan to take forward to your next placement.

✏️ **Notes**

Completion of your practice assessment documentation

You will be required to complete your practice assessment documentation, which may be an online version or paper copy. It is essential there is an ongoing dialogue with your mentor/supervisor regarding your progress and that any issues are highlighted in a timely fashion and addressed in liaison with your university representative. Competencies and achievements in accordance with your university documentation should be completed, and signed by your mentor/supervisor. It can be useful to reflect together with your mentor/supervisor and maximise your learning opportunities. You will also need to document your practice placement hours as part of the NMC requirements.

Notes

By completing a community placement you should discover that you have not only gained confidence due to increased autonomous responsibility, but also a plethora of new or improved transferable skills which can inform your practice for your next placement or nursing career. You will have a greater understanding of community nursing and how the primary and secondary sectors should collaboratively function to promote smooth transitional care of the person/patient involved.

At the end of your placement, you may identify that community nursing is an area of interest to you. If so, consider:

- Making contacts for future networking
- Researching your area of interest and potential opportunities
- Arranging visits to your area of interest
- Arranging shadowing opportunities.

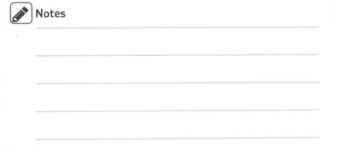 **Notes**

General

Benson, H., Dougherty, L. and McWhirter, A. (2015) Medicines management. Chapter 12 in L. Dougherty and S. Lister (eds) *The Royal Marsden Manual of Clinical Nursing Procedures*, 9th edition. Chichester: Wiley-Blackwell.

Dougherty, L., Lister, S. and West-Oram, A. (2015) *The Royal Marsden Manual of Clinical Nursing Procedures: student edition*, 9th edition. Chichester: Wiley-Blackwell.

#hello my name is... campaign htpp:// hellomynameis.org.uk/

Institute for Healthcare Improvement (2017) SBAR. Available at: bit.ly/IHI-SBAR

McCormack, B. and McCance, T. (2017) *Person-centred Practice in Nursing and Healthcare: theory and practice*, 2nd edition. Chichester: Wiley-Blackwell.

Nursing and Midwifery Council (2007) *Standards for Medicines Management*. London: NMC. Available at: bit.ly/NMC-MED

Nursing and Midwifery Council (2015) *The Code: professional standards of practice and behaviour for nurses and midwives*. London: NMC. Available at: bit.ly/NMC-Code

Oelofsen, N. (2012) *Developing Reflective Practice*. Banbury: Lantern Publishing.

Health visiting

Charity Commission (2014) *Safeguarding Children and Young People*. Available at: bit.ly/SCYP-1

Child Growth Foundation: childgrowthfoundation.org/

Department of Health (2009) *Using the New UK–World Health Organization 0–4 Years Growth Charts*. London: Crown Copyright. Available at: bit.ly/DH-WHO-1

Equality Commission for Northern Ireland (2008) *Every Child an Equal Child*. Available at: bit.ly/ECNI-1 (relates to N. Ireland)

H.M. Government (2003) *Every Child Matters*. Available at: bit.ly/ECM-EW (relates to England and Wales)

Luker, K.A., Orr, J. and McHugh, G.A. (eds) (2012) *Health Visiting: a rediscovery*, 3rd edition. Chichester: Wiley-Blackwell.

Scottish Government (2017) *Getting it Right for Every Child*. Available at: bit.ly/GIRFEC-1 (relates to Scotland)